YOUR KNOWLEDGE HAS VALUE

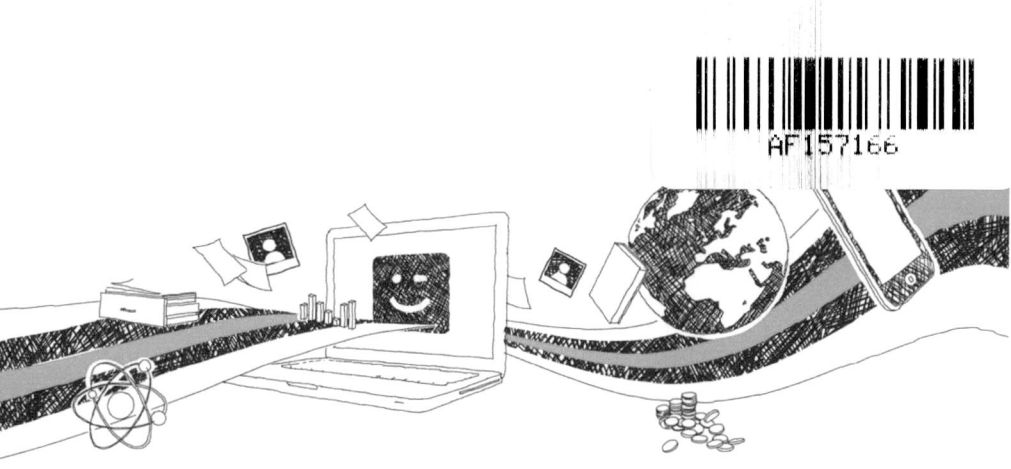
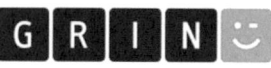

Stephanie Kyle

How does Auditory Processing Disorder Affect Teenagers in their Working Relationships?

GRIN Publishing

Bibliographic information published by the German National Library:

The German National Library lists this publication in the National Bibliography; detailed bibliographic data are available on the Internet at http://dnb.dnb.de .

Imprint:

Copyright © 2012 GRIN Verlag GmbH
Print and binding: Books on Demand GmbH, Norderstedt Germany
ISBN: 978-3-656-94586-4

GRIN - Your knowledge has value

Since its foundation in 1998, GRIN has specialized in publishing academic texts by students, college teachers and other academics as e-book and printed book. The website www.grin.com is an ideal platform for presenting term papers, final papers, scientific essays, dissertations and specialist books.

Visit us on the internet:

http://www.grin.com/

http://www.facebook.com/grincom

http://www.twitter.com/grin_com

How Does APD Affect Teenagers In Their Working Relationships?

Inhaltsverzeichnis

Appendices

Appendices Hand Written
17. Original mind map
18. Second mind map
19. Schedule, 9th February – 30th March
20. Colour coordinated research key
21. Checklist of things to cover in essay

Appendices Doctor's Letters and Handouts Provided By Doctors
22. Dr Nyunt to Dr Maung
24. Dr Nyunt to Miss Bateson
25. ESHV APD advice for schools
26. APD protocol for ESHV involvement
27. Walker Street speech and language therapy service flowchart
28. Activities to minimise the effects of APD (home and school)
29. Strategies to minimise the effects of APD (primary schools)
30. Strategies to minimise the effects of APD (secondary school and beyond)
31. ESHV APD pack
32. "Handy Handout" – suggestions for teachers
33. Booklet – advice for parents and carers
34. Dr Nyunt's APD pack
35. Dr Aung Nyunt Profile

Appendices Survey Results And Emails
36. Email to helpline@ndcs.org.uk, info@deafnessresearch.org.uk, eshv@hullcc.gov.uk
37. Facebook message sent to APD support group
38. Copy of the survey I created and sent

Appendices Internet Research

Appendices Other

Introduction

Imagine how confusing it would be if you are conversing with someone about the economic climate and the person you are liaising with comes out with "the caterpillar was wearing a hat made of yoghurt". Imagine how confusing it would be to pursue a normal day at work and your employer comes up to you and asks you to "sort through the blue trainers and stack them neatly on the lamb shanks". Imagine how confusing it would be if one minute you can understand messages you receive orally and the next minute, words and sentences are completely incomprehensible. It would make you stressed wouldn't it? You would feel stupid and embarrassed when you repeat the sentence for confirmation and the person just laughs at you. You would feel humiliated and insecure.

You are lucky enough to be able to only imagine this situation, however, teenagers with APD unfortunately cannot. This is a reality for them every single day.

APD affects many people across the world for many years of their life, however, not much is known about it. It is sometimes referred to as the "invisible disease". APD is a personal topic that is very close to my heart and very important to me as someone in my family suffers with it. This is the main reason why I have chosen to write my dissertation on APD. I want to raise awareness of it - even if it is only within my college, it will still contribute to the work of charities such as APDUK, ESHV and Deafness Research.

When narrowing down my question from my topic, I took into account all of the different age groups that it affects and my research showed that there is only really support for younger children. This is due to the fact that research has shown that the older the child gets, the less impact APD has on them and they will normally grow out of it by the time they are around 12 years of age. This is not always the case, a lot of people still continue to have it all of their life.

I wanted to focus how APD specifically affects teenagers if they haven't grown out of it. Teenage years are very stressful with all of the important life-changing educational decisions to make. They need to decide which options to choose then which college to go to, next they need to choose their AS Level subjects and which university to go to - essentially, teenagers need to make a choice as to which career path to take from the age of 14. They meet new teachers every year and when at college, are introduced to a whole new system of teacher-student liaison.

Socially, teenagers are under pressure to make friends and then fit in with their new social groups in new classes at the beginning of each secondary school year. When starting at college, they meet new people that they have never even seen before so this is an even more awkward situation for them to be in. This is of course before worrying about being bullied.

Teenagers also participate in work experience at school and/or undertake a part-time job. They are put in new situations with employers, co-workers and customers where they have to develop new styles of communication to suit each person.

Between the ages 13-19, people begin and develop most relationships with all kinds of individuals. This proves more stressful for a teen with APD. By combining all of the above approaches, I decided to investigate into the question "How Does APD Affect Teenagers in Their Working Relationships". In this dissertation, I hope to explore the social, educational and employment associated relationships of a teenager and how APD impacts building and maintaining these connections.

So What Is APD?

APD stands for Auditory Processing Disorder also known as Central Auditory Processing Disorder. At a conference in Texas in April 2000, 14 globally spread senior scientists and clinicians defined APD as being "a deficit in the processing of information that is specific to the auditory modality, that may be exacerbated in unfavourable acoustic environments, and that may be associated with difficulties in listening, speech understanding, language development, and learning." [1]

Each of the human senses have special areas of representation in the brainstem and the brain [2]. The auditory system provides perhaps the most important of those sensory systems since it affords us with a means of verbal communication. A normal Central Auditory Nervous System (CANS) enables us to prioritise certain sounds that are useful to us and it filters out all other sounds. It is then the brain's job to assign a meaning to each of these sounds or auditory stimuli which the ears receive. For example, our brain lets us know that the whistling that we can hear is a bird singing. This process of filtering and attaching a label to relevant auditory stimuli prevents all sounds running together and causing "noise madness". When the above processes do not occur in a person's Central Auditory Nervous System, we call it Auditory Processing Disorder.

When these processes aren't done, it causes a lot of problems in everyday life and especially in building relationships with people.

How Many People Have APD?

Auditory Processing Disorder is a relatively recently recognised condition (first noted in the USA in the mid 1960's) that we do not understand a lot about. It is unknown exactly how many people have it or how they have it but various estimates have been made. According to Kingston Upon Hull's senior APD specialist Dr. Aung Nyunt, approximately 3% of the population of Britain (all ages) have some varying degree of Auditory Processing Difficulties [3], another study estimates that as many as 10% of children may have some level of APD [4] and a child is considered to actually have Auditory Processing Disorder instead of just a difficulty if they fall into the lowest 5 percentile in 2 or more areas of a 3 section assessment [5]. This could imply that up to 0.725% of tested children in Britain have APD although there is not any firm evidence to support this.

Why Do People Have APD?

There have been various studies into why people have APD; all with failure to determine a definite and specific cause of it. There are various categories of causation that have been suggested under which a number of specific etiologic agents could be operating. The most common theory is that a neuromorphologic (nervous system) disorder may account for the majority of people diagnosed with APD [6]. Underlying APD in this group would be areas of polymicrogyri (malformation of the brain) e.g. underdeveloped and misshapen cells as well as misplaced cells, most likely in the left hemisphere and the auditory region of the corpus callosum (also known as the colossal commissure, is a wide, flat bundle of neural fibres beneath the cortex of the brain). Another suggestion is that it is caused by head traumas or certain long-term middle ear diseases such as Glue Ear and severe ear infections [5]. Other possible causes include inheritance [7] and psychological traumas as an infant [8].

How Does APD Affect Working Relationships With Friends?

One of the main effects of APD is that the ears hear things but the brain doesn't understand these sounds. Imagine playing "Chinese whispers", a game where a message is passed on from one person to another and usually ends up nothing like the original sentence. Every sentence that a person with APD hears is like Chinese whispers but backwards and where time replaces each person in the game. The message is completely jumbled and confusing. They may believe they hear something like "Are you going to the four-metre spa?" [9] This happens when the brain struggles to label correctly. Sometimes, the more time that passes, the clearer the phrase becomes and they may then believe they heard "Are you something to tutor something more". The person with APD would obliviously use a procedure called "auditory closure" which is the ability to fill in the missing pieces when parts of a message are not heard or understood, relying on higher-level language and reasoning skills as well as contextual cues [10].

If you have ever assembled a jigsaw puzzle, you know it is much easier if you have a picture to refer to or if you know of what the final assembly is supposed to represent. A similar principle applies to auditory closure abilities. It is far easier to fill in the missing pieces of a message when you have a general idea of what the message is and a good vocabulary from which to choose likely candidates. Sometimes a person with APD can "guess" what the missing words are although; sometimes the words they choose aren't always the right ones.

This proves difficult with every single sentence of every day, however it is even more so when making new friends either at school or college. The inability to interpret words and understand what is being said, people with APD may appear "disinterested" [12], "not very bright" [11] [12] and "rude" [11] [13].

When approaching people to initiate conversation and become acquaintances, at school and college, this is normally in a noisy corridor or recreation area. The inability to filter out background noise makes it difficult to hear what is being said. Auditory closure will probably be used however the noisier it is; the harder it becomes to join a conversation with an understanding of what the topic is. The person with APD could possibly be ridiculed for coming out with something random and off topic and feel very left out. [14] [15] [16] This then results in low self-esteem, and nearly all of these teens will lose confidence and end up feeling insecure; they will repeatedly encounter moments of despair [17] – another reason why people will not want to befriend them.

Even before conversing with others, people will make a judgement of an individual with APD for a number of reasons. Due to difficulties in the classroom, a person with APD will have to catch up a lot outside of school/college therefore; they will be assigned the stereotype of being a "nerd" or "teacher's pet". Unfortunately, those who are classified as being a nerd are most likely to be at the risk of being bullied. Also, APD affects some people in their speech as the brain cannot interpret the words that are being spoken and will distort the way they are presented [4] [18] [19]. These people will also be a bullying target. This means that it will be even more difficult to make friends as others do not want to be friends with those who are bullied as they fear that they will also then be targeted. Also, if other people have low esteem themselves, they like to see other people being bullied and are more likely to join in rather than offer a helping hand.

Time spent studying at home or during free periods at school or college means there is a lot less time for socializing and friends. Friends may feel like the person with APD is ignoring them or avoiding them and even friendships made become strained and due to time restraints, pressure is placed on the relationship and friends grow apart.

Because the brain fails to filter out background noise on a regular basis, someone with APD is most likely to be startled easily and these noises will be stored in the long term memory.

The thing that created the noise will be forever associated with fear hence, the majority of APD sufferers will also have an unusual phobia or phobias relating to the noise. For example, a girl was startled by a flushing toilet cistern and so every time she came across a similar noise, experienced fear. This escalated into Corporophobia (the phobia of toilets in general). [20] Many APD sufferers develop Claustrophobia also.

Possible friends will be put off by the fact that people with APD have crazy phobias. They come across as weird and are again ridiculed. People think they are "psychos" and "idiots" but they just do not understand the problems relating to the condition and do not want to try to understand. [21]

How Does APD Affect Working Relationships With Educators?

An intense curriculum at GCSE and A Level means there is a lot of information to take in for all students in a class. The increasing pressure of attaining satisfactory grades requires remembering and understanding this information. Even the simplest of tasks are a challenge for those with APD.

One way of making coping with APD easier is to liaise in short sentences using only key words [22] [4] as the less words there are in a sentence, the less there is to cause confusion. Teachers cannot do this in a lesson as there is the rest of the class to consider. This usually concludes with the unsuccessful use of auditory closure or the teenager with APD missing out information completely and leaves them confused and distressed. Sometimes, when auditory closure does work in these circumstances, in the amount of time it takes the brain to process the information, the student has missed the following sentence. [22] [23]

With new technologies, teaching tools such as interactive whiteboards are the main focus of the lesson. The only problem is, the teacher will have to face it in order to scribe or manipulate the board hence their face is away from view and their voice is projected in the opposite direction to the student. Because APD can cause a processing delay [24], to an individual with the condition, there can be a constant lag like when a television picture is out of sync with the sound. This can be especially confusing and often nothing at all is understood when this occurs, so some people decide to learn to lip-read to a certain extent to ease this effect. Also, if a person affected by the condition thinks they hear either the word "spoon" or "goon", if they are watching the lip movements of the speaker, they can distinguish which word is being said. This process cannot be carried out properly in a classroom situation if the teacher is not facing the student or is walking around the room [22].

Teachers nowadays also tend to use PowerPoint presentations to provide information but quickly move onto the next slide before a teenager with APD can read through and understand the contents of it. Again, due to the processing delay, this becomes a problem.

In some teenagers, their activity levels may increase because they have to burn up much more energy than average teens in order to pay attention and understand what is being taught in school or college. Other teenagers with APD exhibit lower-than-normal activity levels (hypo activity) [25]. These pupils do not act up in the classroom; in fact, they appear to be either passive, lethargic or reserved. Often parents report that their children are very fatigued after school [25] [26] [27]. They are expending a significant amount of energy just trying to receive auditory information in a meaningful manner as well as the brain burning a lot of energy in concentration and constant studying. They are then very tired in lessons and some teachers who don't understand how APD affects a student's learning may see them as being "lazy" or "not paying attention". If work is not completed during lesson time when information was given out, teachers may expect all pupils to complete the work at home.

The part of the condition that prevents sound discrimination also interferes when reading and memorising. Someone with APD will struggle to read as the brain treats the thinking and reading voice in their head as a separate sound and when there is background noise, this becomes a problem. It can take a number of attempts at reading the same passage to fully comprehend the context it is written in and by the time they have got to the bottom of the page, all knowledge of the previous section has been forgotten [20]. It can take people with APD up to ten times longer to understand the work and complete the tasks involved. This further lowers the self-esteem of APD sufferers and consequently reduces the time for them to work on relationships with friends and family.

Problems can arise in exams because although teenagers with APD are entitled to up to 25% extra time in their exams [32], this time isn't always enough. They can read exam questions wrong several times or have difficulty interpreting the questions, especially if there is background noise such as pencils scribbling, pages turning etc. [32] [33]

The above can cause conflict in relationships with teachers and tutors as the student may come to dislike the teacher for expecting such a lot of work from them which will not be much to another student. This impedes on both their school and home life and can put pressure on other relationships.

The fact that teens with APD are often classified as under-achievers by their teachers [25] does not ease the bridge between teacher and student. It is harder to build a healthy working relationship also, when the teacher does not understand the condition as the student can get angry and frustrated.

Some teens that are having trouble coping with their auditory world "act up because of extreme frustration and confusion [2]. This could be because they feel like nobody understands how they feel and how much of a struggle their life is [28], it could be because the frustration with not being able to do things like others builds up and they just want to be normal [20] or it could be for many other things. A teacher will get angry if a child always forgets what to do or forgets their homework or does a completely different piece of work because they thought the teacher said page XX instead of page XY [29]. Even though the teacher will be aware of the condition, more likely than not, they will snap at the child at some point.

Teenagers are already fairly sensitive at this time in their lives and with the added stress, some teens will have a meltdown and a large number will become cynical, argumentative and even aggressive because of the distress the condition is a causing them [8] [30]. They get easily flustered and frustrated when they cannot accomplish something simple like "normal" people can [25].This can also cause conflict between a teacher and a student as the teacher will not appreciate a teen "playing up" in their lesson.

Disputes with a teacher can also occur when an APD sufferer is positive that the teacher taught the wrong thing. The Central Auditory Nervous System is vast and is also responsible for functions such as attention and converting working memory to short term and then long term storage [31]; however, this is where the condition of APD transpires. This effects the auditory memory conversions in a way that the brain remembers exactly half way through the process of "unravelling what is being said" which is not always correct. This in effect actually alters the auditory memory.

Problems can arise when this happens as an APD sufferer can be absolutely certain they heard one thing when actually this never happened. They can then be accused of lying and this can ignite arguments between teacher and student as well as is social life.

The short term memory is used to process a conversation rather than remember what you have heard. The result of this is that often students with APD will leave a lesson or lecture with no recognition of what they have just been taught as they have not had much extra short term memory available for storage [12]. They will have to do lots of revision after the lesson to keep up with the rest of the class taking up the majority of their time [5].

This constant revision can cause more problems as if the student has misunderstood the material in the first place and then constantly revised the wrong information, they will become frustrated and this could possibly lead to blaming the teacher as there is nowhere else to address anger.

It is not always definite that an educator will be local - some will be from other countries; some will simply be from a different city in the region. APD makes understanding speech a complex process, let alone when the person speaking has a foreign accent. An inability to adapt to a wide variety of speaking styles and enunciations [8] can make understanding people from a different area incredibly difficult and can put stress on an existing or potential relationship as failure to differentiate what is being said can make a conversation awkward. People with APD will possibly have to ask for repetitions numerous amounts of times [31] and the other in conversation may become frustrated. Awkward encounters like these may urge students with APD to avoid particular teachers as the last time they conversed, they felt embarrassed. This would then severely affect the relationship.

Equally, a positive aspect of APD in educational surroundings is that because teenagers diagnosed with APD struggle to express themselves clearly through the use of speech and communication [4][7], their artistic skills are enhanced and a lot of talent is displayed in creative subjects such as art and music [34][35][20]. These are the subjects that APD sufferers normally excel in as well as mathematics in which not much vocabulary is used – just figures.

A common field with an educator will enable opportunities for conversation and the start of a working relationship. Feelings and ideas can be presented through music or art and a teacher specific to this subject can understand and appreciate what is meant without the use of words if necessary. This connection can make a teenager feel respected and accepted and it can build up their confidence knowing they have a teacher who they can rely on. This obviously has a very positive affect on a working relationship and the teenager themselves.

How Does APD Affect Working Relationships With Employers?

Around the ages 15-16, a vast amount of teenagers decide to take up a part time job to earn a little extra money and/or to gain some experience for the future. The first issue for someone with APD is trying to find an employer that is willing to take n someone with special needs. It is unfortunate but true that many people go for jobs and their CV will be more than acceptable, but the minute they inform an employer of a disability in any form, they are no longer required.

The fear of losing a job because of a disability can be very pressurising and stressful and this can result in a poorer performance in the work place. Poor performance means there is more of a chance of being made redundant and the vicious circle repeats. This can either go one of two ways; the employer – employee relationship could be non-existent as both may feel that any encounters would be awkward. It could also be that the employer appears friendly and the relationship would be strong as the employer wants his APD member of staff to feel comfortable and supported. There is also the risk of this relationship being built on patronisation and discriminatory.

There are certain jobs that will be more taxing than others due to memory issues and constant background noise such as waitressing, babysitting, telesales and customer services etc. [39] Defective memory and memory alterations play a huge part in making these jobs an almost impossible task [12] [38].

Again, the main physical element of APD concerns the Central Auditory Nervous System (CANS) and its inability to "label" sounds. A similar dysfunction initiating with the same cause is that the CANS also fails to recognise tone [25]. The result of this is that people with APD can feel like everyone is speaking to them harshly and will take everything literally [36] [12] [37]. Teenagers are known for their mood swings so when the above obstacle is also applied, emotions run riot and leaves them very agitated. Humour with colleagues cannot be carried out successfully as a person with APD cannot understand the sarcasm/intention [37] of the joke and are often referred to as gullible for thinking they were being serious.

This can cause a lot of problems in everyday life but it is particularly distressing in a work environment where there is a hierarchy of authority. Here there is a high chance of being told what you are doing incorrectly and as tone cannot be sensed, teenagers in this situation will become upset and easily perturbed – possibly even aggressive [17]. Professional relationships with employers could be volatile and may result in dismissal if it reaches this extent.

Why Do Some People Choose Not to Tell Others About Their Condition?

The saddening thing about APD is that some people diagnosed with it are too embarrassed to tell friends, employers, or teachers because they are afraid of how they will react. If when trying to create a new friendship you made the other person aware that you have a brain disorder, because of today's society, they will think that you are some form of psycho or that you are dim despite your academic ability in certain subjects. At a job interview, when the interviewer hears that you have a brain disorder that affects your memory and attention span, you will get worked up very easily and you can't understand a word they are saying the majority of the time, it won't go down very well. This is even before they have given you a chance to prove that you are an excellent worker when working in a slightly different style. Teachers will presume you are at the lower ability end of the class and be surprised when you attain an A grade in art or mathematics.

On the other end of the scale, you may be treated in a patronising way. Your boss may only keep you working because it makes them look good on their equal opportunities evaluation or because they pity you, teachers may be condescending and friends may only be your friend because they feel mean if they wasn't seeing as you have a disability.

I have also purchased 2 books on the topic of APD. One of which is written by APD specialist – Teri James Bellis titled "When the Brain Can't Hear", and the other is named "Like Sound through Water" by Karen J. Foli and Edward M. Hallowell which is a personal journey through APD. I also borrowed a book from the Hull University library, a medical book by Gail D. Chermak and Frank E. Musiek called "Central Auditory Processing Disorder – New Perspectives" which was published for medical studies and professional use. These again will have to be specific to numerous publishing acts of the law.

In Conclusion

To answer my original question "How Does APD Affect Teenagers in Their Working Relationships?" I say dramatically.

There is no cure for Auditory Processing Disorder. People learn to adapt to life with the condition, in order to attempt to fit in, in different ways.

APD will affect the lives of every single person that is diagnosed with it as well as anyone relating to them and everybody they become involved with, from friends and family to their dentist. Some people believe that it doesn't affect them one bit, some are even convinced that they don't have a problem. I think this is because they have incorporated APD into their lives and various methods of dealing with it so this is all they have ever known; therefore, to themselves and their family, they are normal. It is only when you have a "bad day" where you are on the verge of a mental breakdown that you realise just how much it does impact your life in every little detail. As the mixed responses from the survey and supporting articles show, every factor of daily routine is controlled by aspects of the condition. Simple things that may seem insignificant to other people are of huge importance to APD sufferers. One example of a method for managing to get through the day is the use of Post-it Notes to remind you to do something, such as have breakfast - even a task that obvious can easily be lost when the CANS attempts to do too many things.

The majority of my research comes from my survey responses however I strongly believe that these people are the only ones who can really judge whether APD affects them or not. After all, they are the ones who have to cope with it on a daily basis.

I know exactly what these people go through to try and be normal, to try and fit in, to be discriminated against, have a bad day, how much extra work is needed to be even close to keeping up with everyone else and how much APD has changed their lives in positive and negative ways. I know this because I was diagnosed with APD in 2007 after my mum battled for a very long time to have my condition diagnosed once and for all.

So, "How Does APD Affect Teenagers In Their Working Relationships?"

An unbelievable amount!

Bibliography

1. J Jerger, F Musiek: Report of the Consensus Conference on the Diagnosis of Auditory Processing Disorders in School-Aged Children. April, 2000
2. http://www.gapacademy.ca/files/CAPDResearchLink.pdf
3. A letter to Dr. M Maung from Dr. Aung Nyunt confirming APD diagnosis. 5th April 2007
4. www.deafnessresearch.org.uk/factsheets.apd.pdf
5. Extract from a hand out given by Educational Services For Hearing And Vision for parents and carers
6. F Musiek, K Gollegly, M Ross: Profiles of types of central auditory processing disorder in children with learning disabilities. J Childhood Comm Disorders 1985
7. An extract from an information pack provided by Dr. A. Nyunt (Hull's APD Specialist)
8. http://www.crisiscounseling.com/articles/capd.htm
9. an example used from http://qw88nb88.wordpress.com/living-with-auditory-processing-disorder/ (a blog of a teenager with APD)
10. When The Brain Can't Hear – Teri Bellis pg. 321, Feb 2002
11. Judith Paton – Adult Audiologist www.judithpaton.com
12. http://qw88nb88.wordpress.com/living-with-auditory-processing-disorder/ (a blog of a teenager with APD)
13. Survey response, anonymous from Boulder, CO, USA. Question 6, 18th Feb 2012 19:37.
14. Survey response, anonymous from Milwaukee, Wisconsin. Question 6, 21st Feb 2012 00:48.
15. Survey response, anonymous from Baton Rouge, LA, USA. Question 6, 23rd Feb 2012 05:42.
16. Survey response, anonymous from Sunnyvale, California, USA. Question 6, 24th Feb 2012 20:16
17. www.crisiscounseling.com/articles/capd.htm
18. Survey response, anonymous from Three Lakes, WI, USA. Question 6, 20th Feb 2012 16:34.
19. Survey response, anonymous from Boulder, CO, USA. Question 6 19th Feb 2012 03:38
20. Interview with Lynne Laverick (mother of APD sufferer)
21. Survey response, anonymous from India. Question 4, 2nd March 2012 06:49.
22. Extract from an Educational Services for Hearing and Vision advice sheet for schools
23. Survey response, anonymous from Alameda, CA, USA. Question 9, 17th Feb 2012 23:41.
24. Royal Berkshire NHS patient information sheet
25. www.gapacademy.ca/files/CAPDResearchLink.pdf
26. Survey response, anonymous from Australia. Question 9, 17th Feb 2012 23:54
27. Survey response, anonymous from Northborough, MA. Question 9, 21st Feb 2012 05:19
28. Survey response, anonymous from Three Lakes, WI, USA. Question 5, 20th Feb 2012 16:33.
29. Survey response, anonymous from Castro Valley, USA, question 9, 23rd Feb 2012 03:42
30. Survey response, anonymous from Sunnyvale, California, USA. Question 9, 24th Feb 2012 20:18
31. American Speech-Language Hearing Association Terminology and definitions sheet.
32. A letter from Dr Aung Nyunt to Miss Bateson SENCO at Andrew Marvell School Concerning extra exam time. 30th Sept 2009
33. Survey response, anonymous from USA, Hudson OH, question 9, 24th Feb 03:11
34. When The Brain Can't Hear - Teri Bellis, pg. xv, Feb 2002
35. When The Brain Can't Hear - Teri Bellis, pg. 102`, Feb 2002
36. Survey response, anonymous from Three Lakes, WI, USA. Question 6, 20th Feb 2012 16:36
37. Survey response, anonymous from Manchester, England. Question 6, 19th Feb 2012 12:45